Table of Contents

Better Bloody Mary: Tomato, Strawberry, Basil

Papaya Creamsicle Smoothie: Papaya, Carrot, Banana

Avo-Cacao Smoothie: Avocado, Peanut Butter, Cacao

Green and Blue: Avocado, Blueberry, Spinach

A.K.C. Champion Smoothie: Avocado, Kiwi, Cucumber

Watermelon Sparkler: Watermelon, Cucumber, Lemon

Lemon Drop Smoothie: Lemon & Cucumber

Sweet Shirley Temple: Cherry, Orange, Ginger

P.B & K: Pineapple, Blueberry, Kale

Purple Power Punch: Red Cabbage, Cherry, Blackberry

Pina Caul-ada-flour Smoothie: Cauliflower, Pineapple, Orange

Hibiscus Citrus Quencher: Hibiscus Tea, Orange, Strawberry

Spiced Orange Smoothie: Orange, Turmeric, Cinnamon

Pineapple Zinger: Pineapple, Ginger

Maximum Mango Smoothie: Mango, Cayenne, Strawberry

Lettuce Be Cherry: Romaine Lettuce, Blueberry, Cherry

The Ultimate Cress: Watercress, Apple, Avocado

Dressed to Dill: Cucumber, Spinach, Dill

Black Forest Cake: Cherry, Banana, Almond

Spiced Carrot Cake: Carrot, Almond, Cinnamon

The Absolute Smoothie: Apple, Banana, Strawberry

Servings: 2

Ingredients

- 1 cup strawberries, halved
- 1 red apple, cored quartered, with skin
- ½ cup apple juice , unsweetened
- 1 banana, peeled
- 4-6 ice cubes

Directions

1.	**Combine ingredients in a blender. Cover and blend until smooth.**

Nutritional Information (per serving)

- Calories 137
- Fat .5 g
- Carbohydrates 34.6 g
- Sugar 18.2 g
- Protein 1 g

Refreshing Classic: Oranges, Apple, Grape

Servings: 2

Ingredients

- 1 red apple, cored and quartered, with skin
- ½ cup apple juice , unsweetened
- 1 orange, peeled and separated
- 1 cup red grapes
- 4-6 ice cubes

Directions

1.   **Combine ingredients in a blender. Cover and blend until smooth.**

Nutritional Information (per serving)

- Calories 303.9
- Fat .4 g
- Carbohydrates 77.9 g
- Sugar 51.4 g
- Protein 2.4 g

Banana Bahama Mama: Banana, Pineapple, Orange

Servings: 2

Ingredients

- 1 cup frozen pineapple chunks, unsweetened
- 1 orange, peeled and separated
- 1 banana, peeled
- ½ cup low-fat vanilla yogurt
- ½ cup coconut water
- 3-5 ice cubes

Directions

1. Combine ingredients in a blender. Cover and blend on high until smooth.

Nutritional Information (per serving)

- Calories 448
- Fat 0 g
- Carbohydrates 51 g
- Sugar 36 g
- Protein 6 g

Orange Power: Orange, Carrot, Turmeric

Servings: 2

Ingredients

- 1 orange, peeled and separated
- 1 ½ cup shredded carrots
- ½ tsp. ground turmeric
- ½ cup water*
- 4-6 ice cubes

Substitute with ½ cup apple juice, if desired.

Directions

1. **Combine ingredients in a blender. Cover and blend until smooth.**

Nutritional Information (per serving)

- Calories 142
- Fat 0 g
- Carbohydrates 35 g
- Sugar 22 g
- Protein 4 g

What a Plummy Pear: Plum, Pear, Blueberry

Servings: 2

Ingredients

- 1 pear, cored and chopped, with skin
- 2 plums, halved and pitted
- 1 cup frozen blueberries, unsweetened
- ½ cup low-fat blueberry yogurt
- ½ tsp. cinnamon

Directions

1.   **Combine ingredients in a blender. Cover and blend until smooth.**

Nutritional Information (per serving)

- Calories 176.3
- Fat 1.6 g
- Carbohydrates 41.5 g
- Sugar 30.9 g
- Protein 2.6 g

Merry Berries and Plum: Cherry, Strawberry, Plum

Servings: 2

Ingredients

- 1 cup strawberries, halved
- 2 plums, pitted and halved
- 1 cup cherries, pitted
- 1 cup original almond milk, unsweetened
- 3-6 ice cubes

Directions

1. **Combine ingredients in a blender. Cover and blend until smooth.**

Nutritional Information (per serving)

- Calories 237
- Fat 3.4 g
- Carbohydrates 54.9 g
- Sugar 42.6 g
- Protein 4.4 g

Apple Pie: Apple, Cinnamon, Almond

Servings: 2

Ingredients

- 2 apples, cored and quartered, with skin
- 2 tbsp. creamy almond butter
- 1 cup original almond milk, unsweetened
- ½ cup low-fat plain yogurt
- ½ tsp. cinnamon
- ¼ tsp. nutmeg
- Pinch cloves
- Pinch of ginger

Directions

1. **Combine ingredients in a blender. Cover and blend until smooth.**

Nutritional Information (per serving)

- Calories 224.7
- Fat 10.6 g
- Carbohydrates 25.9 g
- Sugar 17.2 g
- Protein 10.1 g

Beet the Rush Smoothie: Beet, Strawberry, Raspberry

Servings: 2

Ingredients

- 1 small beetroot, trimmed and quartered
- 1 cup frozen strawberries, unsweetened
- 1 small banana, peeled
- ½ cup red raspberries
- ¾ cup orange juice

Directions

1. **Preheat oven to 400° F.**

2. **While oven is preheating, wash and trim leaves off of beet. Cut into quarters and place on a baking sheet. Bake for 30 minutes, or until soft.**

3. **Combine ingredients in a blender. Cover and blend until smooth.**

Nutritional Information (per serving)

- Calories 146.2
- Fat .8 g
- Carbohydrates 35.5 g
- Sugar 14.4 g
- Protein 2.5 g

Watermelon-Basil Lemonade: Watermelon, Strawberry, Basil

Servings: 2

Ingredients

- 5 cups watermelon, cubed and seeded
- 1 cup frozen strawberries, unsweetened
- ½ cup cucumber slices
- ½ cup lemon juice
- 4 fresh basil leaves

Directions

1. Combine ingredients in a blender. Cover and blend until smooth.

Nutritional Information (per serving)

- Calories 164.2
- Fat 2 g
- Carbohydrates 39 g
- Sugar 28.4 g
- Protein 3.3 g

Creamy Cantaloupe: Cantaloupe, Pineapple, Banana

Servings: 2

Ingredients

- 1 cup cantaloupe chunks
- ½ cup frozen pineapple chunks, unsweetened
- ½ banana, peeled
- ¼ cup shredded carrots
- ½ cup coconut water

Directions

1. **Combine ingredients in a blender. Cover and blend until smooth.**

Nutritional Information (per serving)

- Calories 102
- Fat 0 g
- Carbohydrates 25 g
- Sugar 19 g
- Protein 2 g

Peary-Cherry: Pear, Cherry

Servings: 2

Ingredients

- 1 pear, cored and chopped, with skin
- 1 small apple, cored and quartered, with skin
- 1 cup frozen cherries, pitted
- ½ cup beet juice*
- ½ almond milk, original unsweetened
- 3-5 ice cubes

Substitute with cherry or apple juice , if desired.

Directions

1. **Combine ingredients in a blender. Cover and blend until smooth.**

Nutritional Information (per serving)

- Calories 135.3
- Fat .8 g
- Carbohydrates 33.1 g
- Sugar 21.4 g
- Protein 1.6 g

Peaches and Green: Peach & Avocado

Servings: 2

Ingredients

- 2 ripe peaches, pitted and quartered
- 1 ripe avocado, pitted and peeled
- 1 cup vanilla almond milk, unsweetened
- ½ small banana, peeled
- 1 tbsp. creamy cashew butter*

Substitute with almond or peanut butter, if desired.

Directions

1. **Combine ingredients in a blender. Cover and blend until smooth.**

Nutritional Information (per serving)

- Calories 250.2
- Fat 17.1 g
- Carbohydrates 26 g
- Sugar 12.3 g
- Protein 4.9 g

Sweet Potato Pie: Sweet potato & Banana

Servings: 2

Ingredients

- 1 medium sweet potato
- ½ banana, peeled
- 1 cup vanilla almond milk, unsweetened
- 2 tbsp. creamy cashew butter*
- ½ tsp. cinnamon
- Pinch of nutmeg
- Pinch of ginger
- Pinch of allspice
- 3-4 ice cubes

Substitute with peanut or almond butter, if desired.

Directions

1. **Preheat oven to 350°F.**

2. **While oven is preheating, wash the potato. Pierce several times with a fork before baking it in the oven for 50 minutes, or until tender. Remove peel from potato and cool.**

3. **Once cooled, combine ingredients in a blender. Cover and blend until smooth.**

Nutritional Information (per serving)

- Calories 179.8
- Fat 9.2 g
- Carbohydrates 21.7 g
- Sugar 6.2 g

- Protein 4.7 g

Sweet Peach Tea: Peach, Green Tea

Servings: 2

Ingredients

- 2 ripe peaches, pitted
- 1 cup water
- 1 green tea packet*
- 2 dates, pitted
- 1 small apple, cored and quartered, with skin
- 3-4 ice cubes

Substitute with peach tea, if desired.

Directions

1. Bring 1 cup water to boil, then let cool for approximately 2 minutes, or until 175°F. Steep one green tea packet in water for 1 minute. Remove packet and let cool.

2. Combine ingredients in a blender. Cover and blend until smooth.

Nutritional Information (per serving)

- Calories 139.7
- Fat .3 g
- Carbohydrates 36.2 g
- Sugar 29.1 g
- Protein 1.3 g

Sparkling Peach Spritzer: Peach, Grape

Servings: 2

Ingredients

- ½ cup apple juice
- 1 tbsp. lime juice
- 1 ripe peach, pitted and quartered
- 1 cup seedless green grapes
- 4-5 ice cubes

Directions

1. **Combine ingredients in a blender. Cover and blend until smooth**

Nutritional Information (per serving)

- Calories 107
- Fat .3 g
- Carbohydrates 27.8 g
- Sugar 16.3 g
- Protein 1 g

Cherry Citrus Smoothie: Pineapple, Cherry

Servings: 2

Ingredients

- 1 cup frozen pineapple chunks, unsweetened
- 1 cup cherries, pitted
- ½ cup orange juice
- ½ cup coconut water

Directions

1. **Combine ingredients in a blender. Cover and blend until smooth.**

Nutritional Information (per serving)

- Calories 157
- Fat 0 g
- Carbohydrates 37 g
- Sugar 29 g
- Protein 3 g

Sunrise Smoothie: Kiwi, Watermelon, Strawberry

Servings: 2

Ingredients

- 1 cup watermelon chunks, seedless
- 1 kiwi, peeled and sliced
- ½ cup strawberries, halved
- ½ cup original almond milk, unsweetened
- 4-5 ice cubes

Directions

1. **Combine ingredients in a blender. Cover and blend until smooth.**

Nutritional Information (per serving)

- Calories 64.8
- Fat 1 g
- Carbohydrates 14.6 g
- Sugar 6.7 g
- Protein 1.3 g

Better Birthday Cake: Vanilla, Spinach, Banana

Servings: 2

Ingredients

- ½ banana, peeled
- 1 banana, frozen
- 2 tbsp. creamy cashew butter*
- 1 cup vanilla almond milk, unsweetened
- ½ tsp. pure vanilla extract
- 2 cups spinach

Substitute with almond butter, if desired.

Directions

1. **Combine ingredients in a blender. Cover and blend until smooth.**

Nutritional Information (per serving)

- Calories 214.6
- Fat 9.4 g
- Carbohydrates 30.5 g
- Sugar 16.5 g
- Protein 5.1 g

Blue Raspberry Tea: Blueberry, Raspberry, White Tea

Servings: 2

Ingredients

- 1 cup low-fat blueberry yogurt
- 1 tsp. lemon juice
- 1 cup red raspberries
- 1 cup blueberries
- 1 cup water
- 1 white tea bag
- 3-4 ice cubes

Directions

1. Bring 1 cup water to boil, then let cool for approximately 2 minutes, or until 175°F. Steep one white tea packet in water for 1 minute. Remove packet and let cool.

2. Combine ingredients in a blender. Cover and blend until smooth

Nutritional Information (per serving)

- Calories 120.7
- Fat .3 g
- Carbohydrates 27.4 g
- Sugar 14.4 g
- Protein 4.2 g

Blackberry Mango Tango: Blackberry, Mango, Honeydew

Servings: 2

Ingredients

- 1 cups frozen mango chunks
- 1 cup blackberries
- 1 cup honeydew melon chunks
- 1 cup coconut water
- 1 tsp. pure vanilla extract

Directions

1.   **Combine ingredients in a blender. Cover and blend until smooth.**

Nutritional Information (per serving)

- Calories 108
- Fat 1 g
- Carbohydrates 25 g
- Sugar 16 g
- Protein 2 g

Mango Berry Smoothie: Mango, Blueberry

Servings: 2

Ingredients

- 1 cup blueberries
- 1 cup frozen mango chunks
- 1 cup original almond milk, unsweetened
- 1 tsp lemon juice
- 1 tbsp. raw coconut butter*
- 4-6 ice cubes

Substitute with almond butter, if desired.

Directions

1. **Combine ingredients in a blender. Cover and blend until smooth.**

Nutritional Information (per serving)

- Calories 155
- Fat 7 g
- Carbohydrates 24 g
- Sugar 17 g
- Protein 2 g

You've Broc-To Be Kidding: Broccoli, Blueberry, Orange

Servings: 2

Ingredients

- ¾ cup broccoli florets, de-stemmed
- 2 cups water
- 1 cup blueberries
- 1 orange, peeled and separated
- 1 cup orange juice
- 3-4 ice cubes

Directions

1. In a medium sauce pan, bring water to a boil. Boil broccoli for 7 minutes, or until tender. Remove from heat, drain, and let cool.

2. Combine ingredients in a blender. Cover and blend until smooth.

Nutritional Information (per serving)

- Calories 146.7
- Fat .6 g
- Carbohydrates 34.6 g
- Sugar 25.5 g
- Protein 3.5 g

Blackberry Cobbler: Blackberry, Almond

Servings: 2

Ingredients

- 1 ½ cups blackberries
- ½ cup original almond milk, unsweetened
- 2 tbsp. creamy almond butter
- ½ cup low-fat vanilla yogurt
- 1 tsp. cinnamon
- 1 tsp. vanilla extract
- 4-6 ice cubes
- Optional: add 1 Tbsp. raw honey for a sweeter smoothie

Directions

1. **Combine ingredients in a blender. Cover and blend until smooth.**

Nutritional Information (per serving)

- Calories 166.9
- Fat 9.1 g
- Carbohydrates 20.1 g
- Sugar 10.1 g
- Protein 4.3 g

Lean, Mean, and Green: Spinach, Celery, Kiwi

Servings: 2

Ingredients

- 2 cups spinach
- 2 celery stalks, chopped
- 1 kiwi, peeled
- 1 cup apple juice
- 4-6 ice cubes

Directions

1. **Combine ingredients in a blender. Cover and blend until smooth.**

Nutritional Information (per serving)

- Calories 96.5
- Fat .3 g
- Carbohydrates 22. 7g
- Sugar 14.1 g
- Protein 1.5 g

P. B. & Green: Banana, Peanut butter, Spinach

Servings: 2

Ingredients

- 1 large banana, peeled
- 2 tbsp. creamy peanut butter
- 2 cups spinach
- ½ low-fat yogurt, plain
- ½ cup original almond milk, unsweetened
- 4-6 ice cubes

Directions

1. **Combine ingredients in a blender. Cover and blend until smooth.**

Nutritional Information (per serving)

- Calories 172.3
- Fat 9 g
- Carbohydrates 21 g
- Sugar 10.3 g
- Protein 5.6 g

Very Berry Cranberry: Raspberry, Cranberry

Servings: 2

Ingredients

- 1 cup frozen cranberries
- ½ cup raspberries
- 1 small banana, peeled
- ½ cup original almond milk, unsweetened
- 2 tbsp. orange juice
- 4-6 ice cubes

Directions

1. **Combine ingredients in a blender. Cover and blend until smooth.**

Nutritional Information (per serving)

- Calories 127
- Fat 1 g
- Carbohydrates 28 g
- Sugar 15 g
- Protein 2 g

Feel the Beet: Banana & Beet

Servings: 2

Ingredients

- 1 medium banana, peeled
- 1 small beetroot
- 1 cup vanilla almond milk, unsweetened
- 1 tbsp. creamy peanut butter
- 3-4 ice cubes

Directions

1. **Preheat oven to 400° F.**

2. **While oven is preheating, wash and trim leaves off of beet. Cut into quarters and place on a baking sheet. Bake for 30 minutes, or until soft.**

3. **Combine ingredients in a blender. Cover and blend until smooth.**

Nutritional Information (per serving)

- Calories 132.8
- Fat 5.5 g
- Carbohydrates 19.4 g
- Sugar 10.8 g
- Protein 3.5 g

Super Booster Smoothie: Cranberry, Blueberry, Kale

Servings: 2

Ingredients

- 1 cup kale, raw and chopped
- 1 cup cranberry juice , unsweetened
- 1 cup frozen blueberries, unsweetened
- ½ banana, peeled
- 2 tbsp. orange juice

Directions

1.　　Combine ingredients in a blender. Cover and blend until smooth.

Nutritional Information (per serving)

- Calories 158.2
- Fat 1 g
- Carbohydrates 238 g
- Sugar 29.3 g
- Protein 2.3 g

Cauli-berry Smoothie: Strawberry, Cherry, Cauliflower

Servings: 2

Ingredients

- 1 cup cauliflower florets, de-stemmed
- 1 cup strawberries, halved
- 1 cup frozen cherries, pitted and unsweetened
- 1 small banana
- ½ cup low-fat plain yogurt
- 1 cup original almond milk, unsweetened

Directions

1. Combine ingredients in a blender. Cover and blend until smooth.

Nutritional Information (per serving)

- Calories 170
- Fat 1.8 g
- Carbohydrates 36.5 g
- Sugar 22.7 g
- Protein 6 g

Pumpkin Pie Smoothie: Pumpkin, Banana, Cinnamon

Servings: 2

Ingredients

- 1 cup pumpkin chunks*
- 1 banana
- 1 cup low-fat vanilla yogurt
- 1 tbsp. peanut butter
- 1 tsp. cinnamon
- Pinch of nutmeg
- Pinch of cloves
- 3-4 ice cubes
- Optional: tbsp. pure maple syrup
- Optional: ¼ cup pumpkin seeds

Substitute with 1 cup pumpkin puree, if desired

Directions

1. Preheat oven to 375°F. Bake pumpkin chunks for 50 minutes, or until soft. Peel and let cool.

2. Combine ingredients in a blender. Cover and blend until smooth.

Nutritional Information (per serving)

- Calories 212.1
- Fat 4.3 g
- Carbohydrates 33.6 g

- Sugar 21.7 g
- Protein 11.7 g

Better Bloody Mary: Tomato, Strawberry, Basil

Servings: 2

Ingredients

- 1 cup strawberries, halved
- 2 celery stalks, chopped
- ¾ cup tomato juice , unsalted
- ¼ cup water
- 3-4 basil leaves*
- 1 tsp. lemon juice
- 1/8 tsp. ground black pepper
- Pinch of cayenne pepper
- 4-6 ice cubes
- Optional: 2 celery sticks for garnish

Substitute 2 tbsp. dried basil, if desired

Directions

1. **Combine ingredients in a blender. Cover and blend until smooth.**

2. **Optional: pour and garnish with celery sticks.**

Nutritional Information (per serving)

- Calories 45
- Fat .4 g
- Carbohydrates 10.7 g
- Sugar 7.2 g
- Protein 1.5 g

Papaya Creamsicle Smoothie: Papaya, Carrot, Banana

Servings: 2

Ingredients

- 1 cup papaya, seeded and peeled
- 1 small banana, peeled
- ½ cup shredded carrots
- 1 cup coconut water
- 2 tbsp. orange juice
- 4-6 ice cubes
- Optional: 1-2 dates for a sweeter smoothie

Directions

1. Combine papaya and water; blend. Add banana, carrots, and ice. Cover and blend until smooth.

Nutritional Information (per serving)

- Calories 147.3
- Fat .5 g
- Carbohydrates 34.5 g
- Sugar 23.7 g
- Protein 2.3 g

Avo-Cacao Smoothie: Avocado, Peanut Butter, Cacao

Servings: 2

Ingredients

- 1 avocado, pitted and skinned
- 2 ½ tbsp. raw cacao powder
- 1 banana, peeled
- ½ cup low-fat vanilla yogurt
- 3 tbsp. creamy peanut butter
- ¼ cup vanilla almond milk, unsweetened
- 3-4 ice cubes

Directions

1. **Combine ingredients in a blender. Cover and blend until smooth.**

Nutritional Information (per serving)

- Calories 386.5
- Fat 24.5 g
- Carbohydrates 335.9 g
- Sugar 15 g
- Protein 12.5 g

Green and Blue: Avocado, Blueberry, Spinach

Servings: 2

Ingredients

- 1 ½ cup frozen blueberries, unsweetened
- 2 cups spinach
- 1 small avocado, pitted and peeled
- 1 cup original almond milk, unsweetened
- Pinch of cinnamon
- 3-6 ice cubes

Directions

1. **Combine ingredients in a blender. Cover and blend until smooth.**

Nutritional Information (per serving)

- Calories 206.2
- Fat 13.4 g
- Carbohydrates 23.7 g
- Sugar 9.9 g
- Protein 4.3 g

A.K.C. Champion Smoothie: Avocado, Kiwi, Cucumber

Servings: 2

Ingredients

- ½ avocado, pitted and peeled
- ½ cup apple juice
- 1 cup spinach
- 1 kiwi, peeled
- ½ cup cucumber slices
- 4-6 ice cubes

Directions

1. **Combine ingredients in a blender. Cover and blend until smooth.**

Nutritional Information (per serving)

- Calories 122.5
- Fat 5.9 g
- Carbohydrates 17.9 g
- Sugar 7.1 g
- Protein 2.2 g

Watermelon Sparkler: Watermelon, Cucumber, Lemon

Servings: 2

Ingredients

- 1 cup watermelon chunks, seedless
- ½ cup cucumber slices
- ½ cup green grapes
- 1 tbsp. lemon juice
- 2-3 mint leaves
- 4-6 ice cubes

Directions

1. Combine ingredients in a blender. Cover and blend until smooth.

Nutritional Information (per serving)

- Calories 57.5
- Fat .4 g
- Carbohydrates 14.3 g
- Sugar 11.1 g
- Protein 1 g

Lemon Drop Smoothie: Lemon & Cucumber

Servings: 2

Ingredients

- 1 cup low-fat vanilla yogurt
- ½ cup coconut milk, unsweetened
- ½ cup cucumber slices
- 2 tbsp. lemon juice
- 1 date, pitted*
- 4-6 ice cubes

Substitute 1 tbsp. raw honey, if desired.

Directions

1.	**Combine ingredients in a blender. Cover and blend until smooth.**

Nutritional Information (per serving)

- Calories 102
- Fat 2.7 g
- Carbohydrates 15.8 g
- Sugar 10 g
- Protein 5.5 g

Sweet Shirley Temple: Cherry, Orange, Ginger

Servings: 2

Ingredients

- 1 cup cherries, pitted
- 1 cup orange juice
- 1 small banana
- 1 tbsp. fresh grated ginger*
- 4-6 ice cubes
- Optional: cherries for garnish

Substitute with 1 tbsp. candied ginger, if desired.

Directions

1. **Combine ingredients in a blender. Cover and blend until smooth.**

2. **Optional: Pour and garnish with cherries on top.**

Nutritional Information (per serving)

- Calories 149.3
- Fat .8 g
- Carbohydrates 36.5 g
- Sugar 20.3 g
- Protein 2.3 g

P.B & K: Pineapple, Blueberry, Kale

Servings: 2

Ingredients

- 1 cup kale, chopped
- 1 cup blueberries
- 1 cup frozen pineapple chunks, unsweetened
- 1 cup low-fat blueberry yogurt
- 4-6 ice cubes

Directions

1. **Combine ingredients in a blender. Cover and blend until smooth.**

Nutritional Information (per serving)

- Calories 211
- Fat 2 g
- Carbohydrates 45 g
- Sugar 32 g
- Protein 6 g

Purple Power Punch: Red Cabbage, Cherry, Blackberry

Servings: 2

Ingredients

- 1 cup frozen cherries, pitted
- 1 cup strawberries, halved
- ½ cup blackberries
- 1 cup red cabbage, chopped
- ½ cup juice orange juice
- 1 cup low-fat blueberry yogurt

Directions

1.   **Combine ingredients in a blender. Cover and blend until smooth.**

Nutritional Information (per serving)

- Calories 247.7
- Fat 2.7 g
- Carbohydrates 53.5 g
- Sugar 41.7 g
- Protein 5.3 g

Pina Caul-ada-flour Smoothie: Cauliflower, Pineapple, Orange

Servings: 2

Ingredients

- ½ cup cauliflower florets, de-stemmed
- 1 ½ cup frozen pineapple chunks, unsweetened
- 1 cup coconut milk, unsweetened
- Optional: 2 pineapple wedges for garnish

Directions

1.   Combine all ingredients in a blender. Cover and blend until smooth.

2.   Optional: pour into glasses and garnish the rims with pineapple wedges.

Nutritional Information (per serving)

- Calories 89
- Fat 3 g
- Carbohydrates 17 g
- Sugar 11 g
- Protein 1 g

Hibiscus Citrus Quencher: Hibiscus Tea, Orange, Strawberry

Servings: 2

Ingredients

- 1 cup water
- 1 hibiscus tea bag
- 1 cup frozen strawberries, unsweetened
- 1 orange, peeled and separated
- 1 tsp. cinnamon
- Pinch of black pepper
- 4-6 ice cubes

Directions

1. Heat water to a boil then remove from heat. Steep hibiscus tea bag for 3-5 minutes. Remove bag and let cool.

2. Combine ingredients in a blender. Cover and blend until smooth.

Nutritional Information (per serving)

- Calories 56.8
- Fat .1 g
- Carbohydrates 14.5 g
- Sugar 9.6 g
- Protein .9 g

Spiced Orange Smoothie: Orange, Turmeric, Cinnamon

Servings: 2

Ingredients

- 2 oranges, peeled and separated
- 1 cup cantaloupe chunks, peeled
- 1 cup original almond milk, unsweetened
- ½ tsp. turmeric powder
- ½ tsp. freshly grated ginger
- ½ tsp. cinnamon
- 4-6 ice cubes

Directions

1.   **Combine ingredients in a blender. Cover and blend until smooth.**

Nutritional Information (per serving)

- Calories 103.6
- Fat 1.5 g
- Carbohydrates 16.4 g
- Sugar 18.7 g
- Protein 2.3 g

Pineapple Zinger: Pineapple, Ginger

Servings: 2

Ingredients

- 1 cup frozen pineapple, unsweetened
- 1 small banana, peeled
- 1 tbsp. freshly grated ginger
- ½ cup low-fat peach yogurt
- ½ cup coconut water
- Pinch of cinnamon

Directions

1. **Combine ingredients in a blender. Cover and blend until smooth.**

Nutritional Information (per serving)

- Calories 210
- Fat 7 g
- Carbohydrates 49 g
- Sugar 25 g
- Protein 2 g

Maximum Mango Smoothie: Mango, Cayenne, Strawberry

Servings: 2

Ingredients

- 1 cup mango chunks, peeled
- ½ cup frozen strawberries, unsweetened
- 1 banana, peeled
- ¼ tsp. cayenne pepper
- Pinch of cinnamon
- Dash of lime juice
- Optional: 1 tbsp. raw honey for additional sweetness

Directions

1. **Combine ingredients in a blender. Cover and blend until smooth.**

Nutritional Information (per serving)

- Calories 102.8
- Fat .4 g
- Carbohydrates 26.7 g
- Sugar 18.9 g
- Protein 1 g

Lettuce Be Cherry: Romaine Lettuce, Blueberry, Cherry

Servings: 2

Ingredients

- 1 cup romaine lettuce, chopped
- ½ cup cherries, pitted
- 1 cup blueberries
- 1 cup cherry juice
- 4-6 ice cubes

Directions

1. **Combine ingredients in a blender. Cover and blend until smooth.**

Nutritional Information (per serving)

- Calories 157.4
- Fat .1 g
- Carbohydrates 38.7 g
- Sugar 28.1 g
- Protein 2.3 g

The Ultimate Cress: Watercress, Apple, Avocado

Servings: 2

Ingredients

- ¼ cup watercress
- ½ small avocado, pitted and peeled
- 1 small banana, peeled
- 1 apple, cored and quartered, with skin
- 1 cup apple juice , unsweetened
- 3-6 ice cubes

Directions

1.	**Combine ingredients in a blender. Cover and blend until smooth.**

Nutritional Information (per serving)

- Calories 185
- Fat 6 g
- Carbohydrates 34.9 g
- Sugar 10.5 g
- Protein 2 g

Dressed to Dill: Cucumber, Spinach, Dill

Servings: 2

Ingredients

- 2 cups cucumber slices
- ¼ cup lemon juice
- 5 sprigs of dill
- 1 cup spinach
- 1 cup low-fat plain yogurt
- 4-6 ice cubes

Directions

1. **Combine ingredients in a blender. Cover and blend until smooth.**

Nutritional Information (per serving)

- Calories 1oo.5
- Fat 2.2 g
- Carbohydrates 14 g
- Sugar 8.7 g
- Protein 7.7 g

Black Forest Cake: Cherry, Banana, Almond

Servings: 2

Ingredients

- ½ cup spinach
- 2 small bananas, peeled
- 2 tbsp. creamy almond butter
- 1/3 cup frozen cherries, pitted and unsweetened
- 1 cup vanilla almond milk, unsweetened
- 2 tbsp. raw cacao powder, extra for garnish
- 1 tsp. cinnamon
- 1 tsp. pure vanilla extract
- 3-5 ice cubes
- Optional: fresh cherries for garnish

Directions

1. **Combine ingredients in a blender. Cover and blend until smooth.**

2. **Optional: pour into glasses and garnish with a light dusting of cacao powder and fresh cherries.**

Nutritional Information (per serving)

- Calories 225.9
- Fat 11 g
- Carbohydrates 29.9 g
- Sugar 13.6 g
- Protein 5.5 g

Spiced Carrot Cake: Carrot, Almond, Cinnamon

Servings: 2

Ingredients

- 2 small bananas
- 1 cup shredded carrots
- 1 cup vanilla almond milk, unsweetened
- 2 tbsp. creamy almond butter
- ½ tsp cinnamon
- Pinch of powdered ginger
- Pinch of nutmeg
- Optional: 1 tbsp. raw honey for a sweeter smoothie
- 4-6 ice cubes

Directions

1. **Combine ingredients in a blender. Cover and blend until smooth.**

Nutritional Information (per serving)

- Calories 210.4
- Fat 10.5 g
- Carbohydrates 28.2 g
- Sugar 13.4 g
- Protein 4.4 g

Your Reviews are greatly appreciated, and your experiences help others cope with their own. Please do share your experiences, and help others.

More educational, & diet books on gout & inflammation that you may find helpful.

Click onto each image, and be taken directly to the product page, on Amazon.

Join our Gout & Inflammation Relief newsletter by clicking here: **Join us here**

Other types of great recipe ideas here!

ANTI INFLAMMATION GUIDE

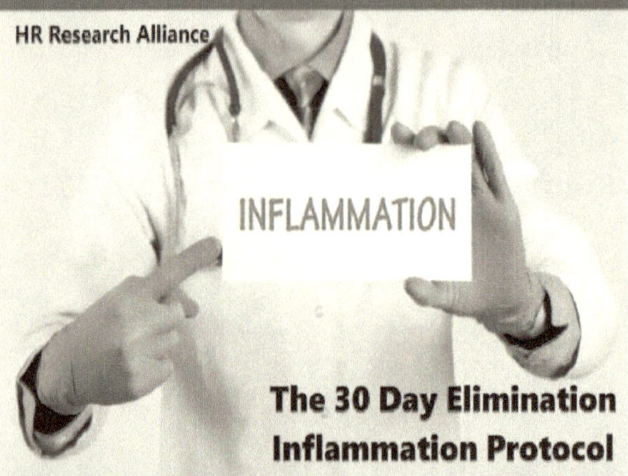

The 30 Day Elimination Inflammation Protocol

Anti Inflammatory Foods - Lifestyle Changes - Tips - Anti Inflammation Cooking - Daily - Weekly - Meal Plans - & More...

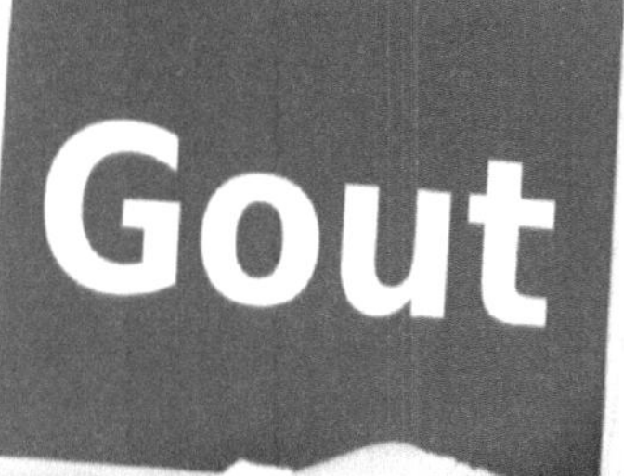
Everything You Must
Know About Gout

HR Research Alliance

Gout

The Ultimate Guide

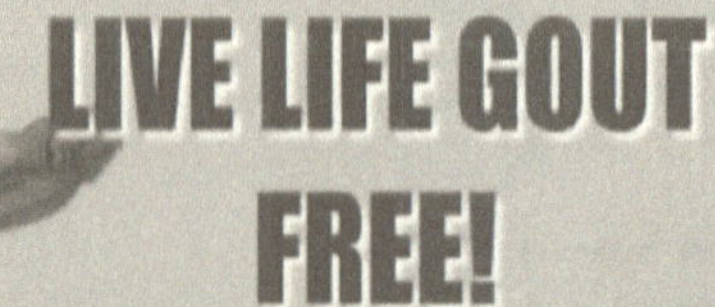

LIVE LIFE GOUT FREE!

GOUT REMEDIES ARE THROUGH DIET

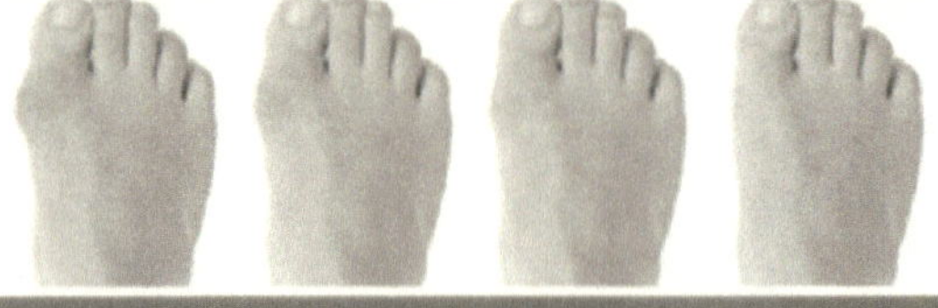

THE ULTIMATE GOUT COOKBOOK - 50 RECIPES FOR INFLAMMATORY RELIEF
GOUT BE GONE
HR RESEARCH ALLIANCE

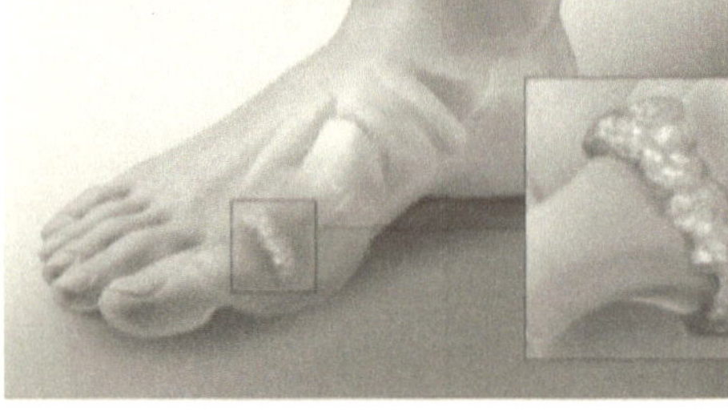

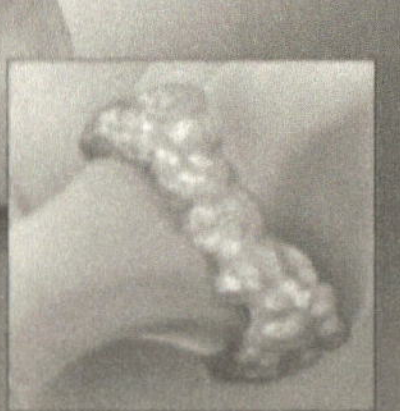

Gout

&

ANTI INFLAMMATION MEAL PLAN GUIDE

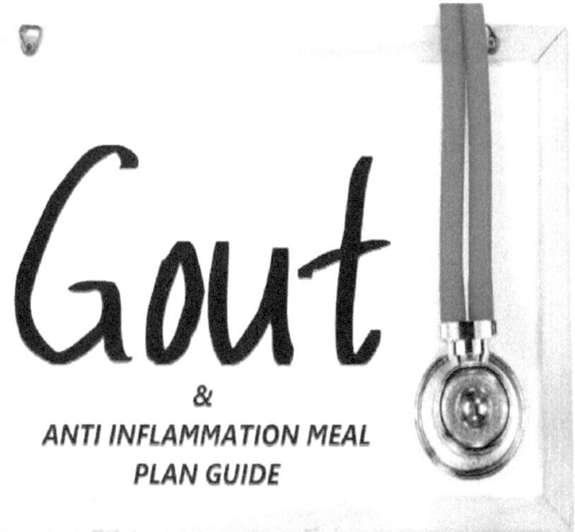

Nutritional Strategies For Reducing Inflammation Naturally

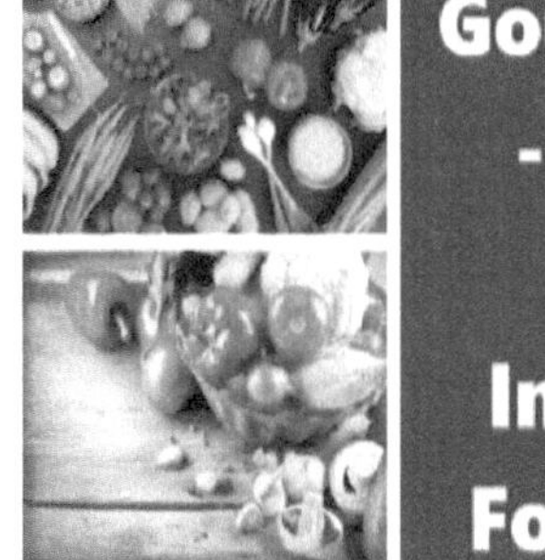

HR Research
Alliance

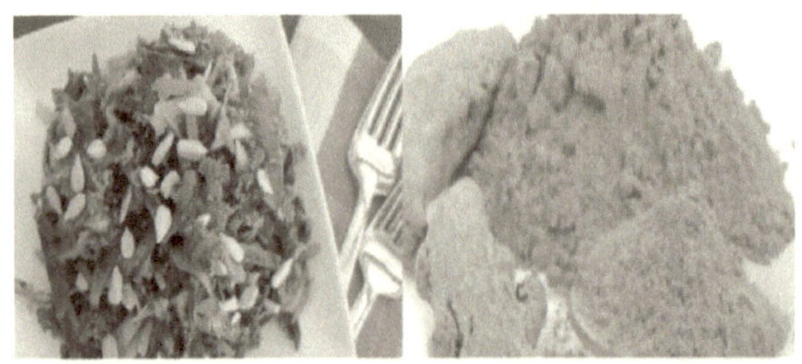

A N T I - INFLAMMATORY

C O O K B O O K

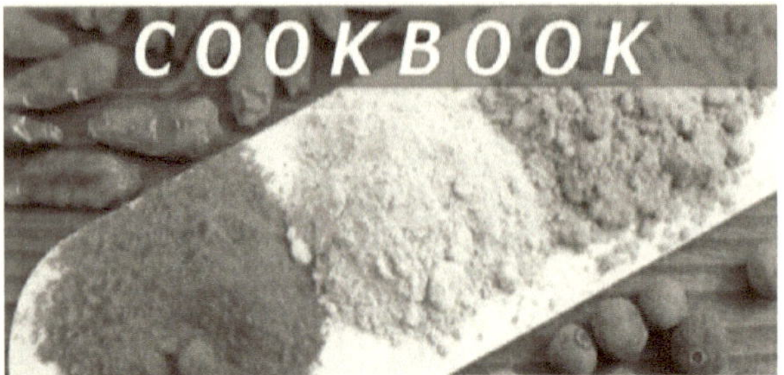

50
Slow Cooker Recipes With Anti - Inflammatory Ingredients

GREAT FOR GOUT RELIEF!

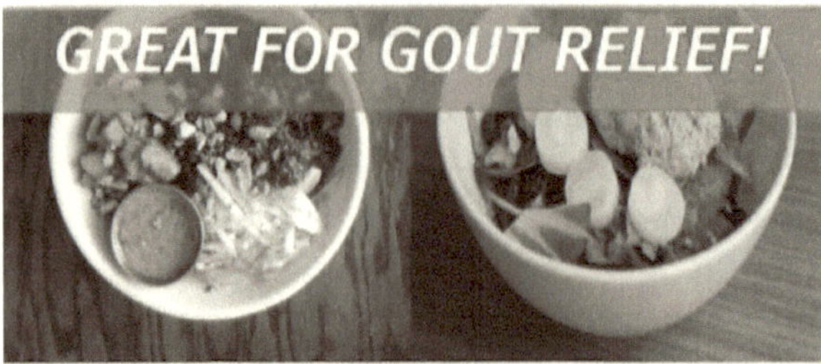

ANTI INFLAMMATION

The Guide To Reducing Inflammation

JT Thorpe

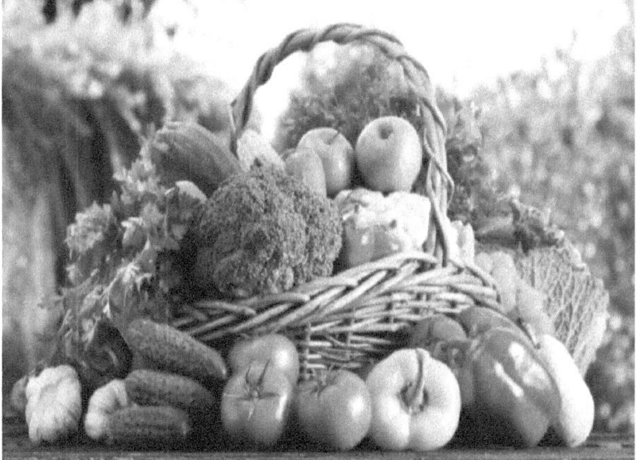

7 Day Meal Plan - Anti Inflammatory Recipes - Lifestyle Changes - How To Reduce Inflammation Naturally - What To Eat - What To Avoid Eating - & Much More Motivational & Useful Information

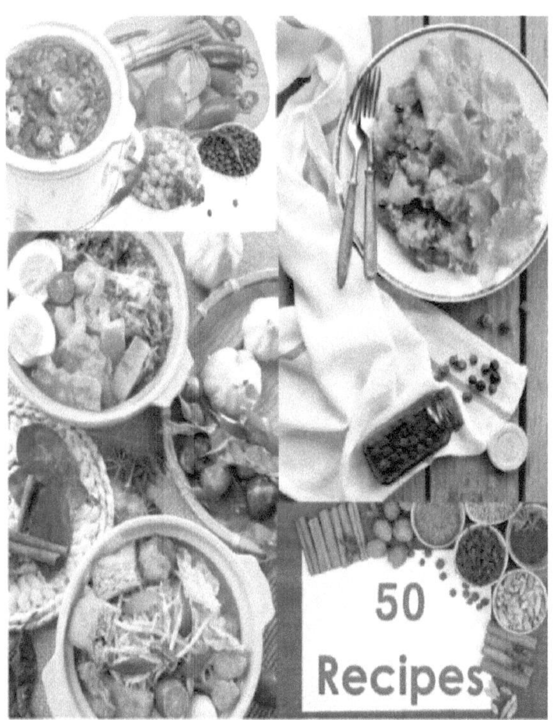

GOUT RELIEF
RECIPES
Kelly Bird

Top 50 Seasoning Recipes

Olivia Rose / Recipe Junkies

The Best
SPICE MIX
RECIPES

Gout Treatment
Gout Diet
GOUT
Prevention

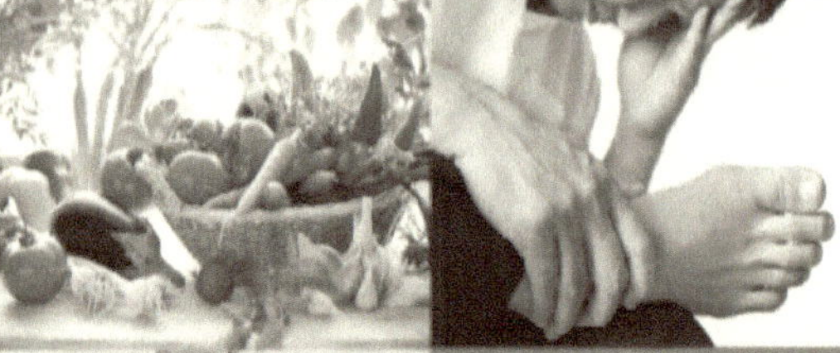

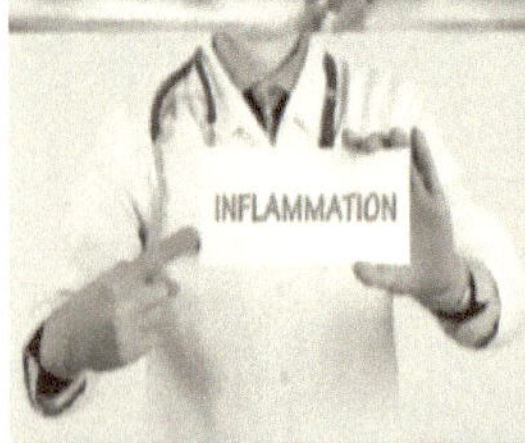

INFLAMMATION

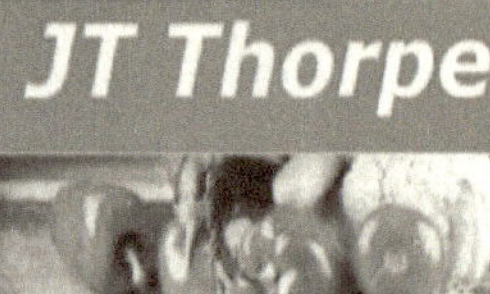

JT Thorpe
Gout Relief

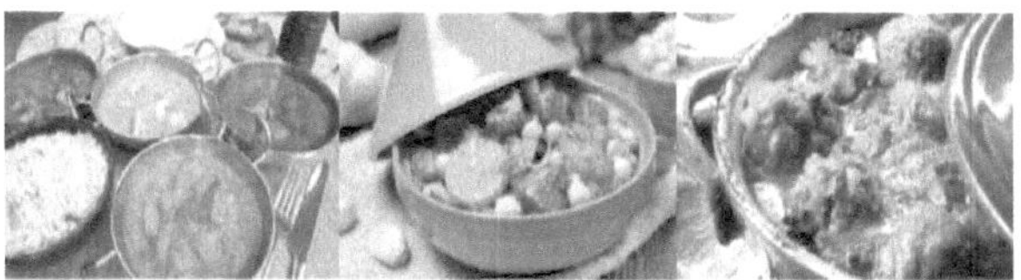

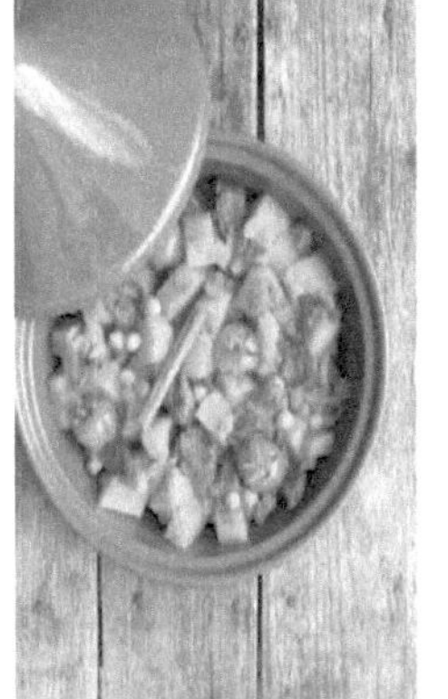

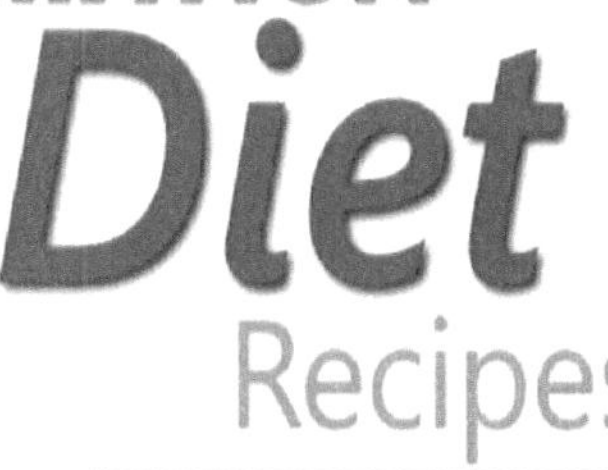

Great For Gout Relief!

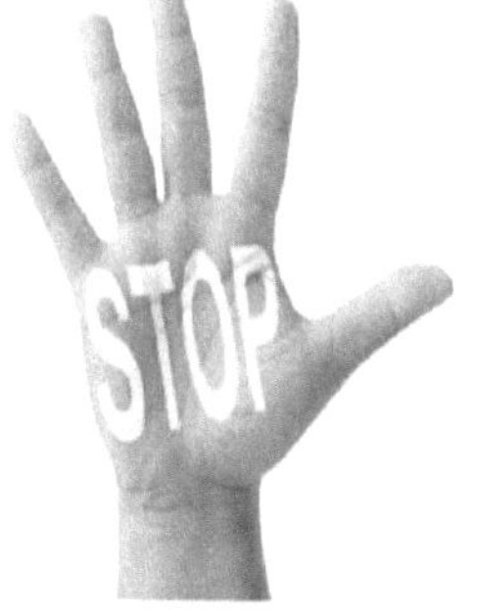

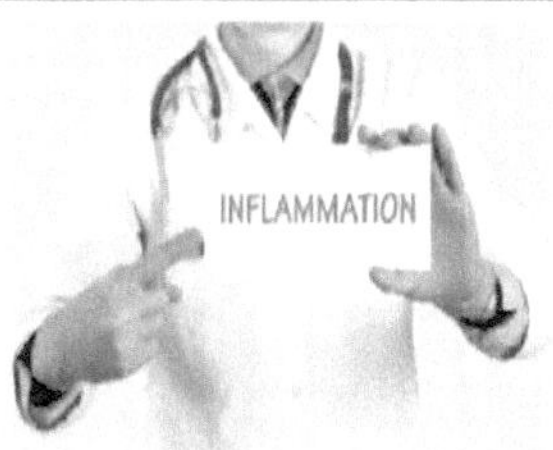

Bonus: GOUT Information

A disease that affects 1 in 100 people, over 1% of the world's total population, which was first diagnosed as early as 2640 BC is most commonly known as Gout.[1, 2] Historically, Gout was referred to with a variety of other names depending on the body part in which it was located such as Podagra (foot), Gonagra (knees) and Chiagra (hands).[3]   Due to links to individuals with a rich diet and excessive alcohol use, Gout has also been nick-named as the "disease of kings".[4]   Hippocrates, a Greek physician known as the father of Western medicine, coined Gout with the phrase of "the unwalkable disease" in the fifth century BC.[2, 5]

So, you may be asking yourself, what is Gout? Plain and simple, it is an inflammatory arthritis which is considered to be one of the most painful forms currently known to mankind. The often sudden and painful inflammation is caused by needle-like crystals that form in joints and/ or soft tissues around the joints as a result of excessive buildup of uric acid.[6] An excess of uric acid takes place when there is an increase in the normal production levels of the breakdown of purines or when the body does not eliminate enough of the acid through the kidneys in the form of urine.[7] When this occurs a condition called hyperuricemia develops in the blood which can cause an excess of uric acid crystals to form thus potentially causing Gout to develop.[7]

When a person has elevated levels of uric acid and there are no other symptoms presented, it is known as Asymptomatic Gout. This is possibly the first of the four stages of Gout; however, it does not usually require any form of treatment.

The next stage is known as Acute Gout and usually leads to sudden swollen joints and intense pain resulting from the formation of the uric acid crystals described previously. The most common time this phase occurs is at night and may be linked to the use of alcohol or drugs, experiencing a period of intense stress or suffering from another illness. Whether or not treatment is administered throughout this phase, the inflammatory attack can last anywhere from a few days to nearly two weeks.

The period of time after an incidence of Acute Gout occurs is known as Intercritical Gout. During this phase there are not any symptoms. Another episode of Acute Gout may not occur for several months or years, but with each attack they can last a longer period of time and take place more often.

The last of the four phases of this disease is known as Chronic Tophaceous Gout and it is considered to be the most disabling stage. Most people do not progress to this stage if they have received proper medical treatment. Those that do enter into this stage may experience permanent damage to their kidneys and / or joints from the long term effects of this disease over the course of 10 or more years.[8]

With nearly 73 million people worldwide affected by Gout, who is most at risk? Those with a family history of the disease are definitely susceptible to it; however, estimates range from 20% - 80% of those with the disease have another member of their family that suffered from the disease. That is a very wide range so we need to gain a clearer understanding beyond genetics to answer this question. Individuals that are most at risk include those that are overweight, drink excessive amounts of alcohol, consume significant foods that are rich in purines, have been exposed environmentally to lead, have certain medical conditions or those that take certain medications. Additionally, men between 40 and 50 years of age and adults over 20 are more at risk than pre-menopausal women and children respectively.[9]

The most common medical conditions included in the at-risk list are individuals with renal insufficiencies, high blood pressure, underactive thyroid glands, psoriasis, anemia and some cancers. Kelley-Seegmiller Syndrome and Lesch-Nyhan Syndrome are two rare medical conditions that are also included on the most at risk listing.[9]

Medications such as diuretics, salicylate-containing drugs such as aspirin, Niacin, Cyclosporine and Levodopa which is used to treat Parkinson's disease are known to increase the risk of both hyperuricemia and gout.[9]

All of the cells within a person's body contain the natural substance known as purines. Additionally, purines provide a portion of the chemical structure of all plant and animal genes which means that virtually all foods will contain them.[10] Those individuals that have been diagnosed with any phase of gout could benefit by avoiding excessive amounts of alcohol and reducing the consumption of foods with high concentrations of purines to help in minimizing future occurrences and symptoms. It is important to acknowledge that diet alone will not prevent or cause gout.

According to the Mayo Clinic the foods that a gout sufferer should eat and avoid are very similar to the recommendations made for anyone to have a healthy and balanced diet. Some of those recommendations include eating more fruits, vegetables and whole grains while avoiding white bread, cakes, candy, sugar-sweetened beverages and products with high-fructose corn syrup. Drinking eight to sixteen 8-ounce glasses of fluids per day with at least half of it being water keeps a person hydrated and has been known to reduce the number of gout attacks. Reducing red meats, fatty poultry and high-fat dairy products in turn reduces the intake of saturated fats. Additionally, it is also recommended to eat no more than four to six ounces of proteins from lean meat, fish and poultry and adding additional proteins from low-fat or fat-free dairy products.[11]

Although vegetables such as asparagus, spinach, peas, cauliflower and mushrooms contain highly concentrated levels of purines, studies have shown that they do not increase the risk of gout or increasing the number of gout attacks. Likewise, beans or lentils have moderately high levels of purines but they are a great source of protein and thus do not need to be avoided.

Supplements to your daily routine such as adding 500-mg of Vitamin C, consuming a moderate amount of regular caffeinated coffee and eating cherries has been known to help reduce the risk of gout attacks and / or reduce uric acid levels within one's body. Prior to taking Vitamin C supplements or drinking coffee should be discussed with a doctor because with certain medical conditions these items may cause other issues or interfere with other medications being taken by the patient.

Those individuals that are in the at-risk group for hyperuricemia and gout or have been diagnosed with one of the phases of gout should avoid organ and glandular meats, red meats, meat extracts, certain types of seafood and yeast products. Examples of organ and glandular meats include liver and kidney. Beef, pork and lamb are examples of red meats to avoid. Meat based soup, broth and gravy are considered meat extracts while beer and baked goods are examples of yeast products. Anchovies, sardines, herring, fish roe, canned tuna fish, shrimp, lobster, scallops and mussels are seafood that contains high levels of purine.

Some of the medications that a physician may prescribe to avoid gout flare-ups may include febuxostat (Uloric), allopurinol (Aloprim, Lopurin, Zyloprim), colchicine (Colcrys) or probenecid (Probalan). According to WebMD, it is very important that a patient taking any of these medications understands that in the first few months of beginning them that a gout attack may still flare-up. Flare-ups may still happen as a result of the patient's body is adjusting to being on the medication and does not mean that the medication does not work. The physician will likely prescribe a specific medicine for these flare-ups to take when they occur in addition to the preventative medication. Adjustments may need to be made with the dosage of the preventative medication in the event that attacks begin occurring after a long period of time taking it.[12]

In order to gain some symptom relief there are some non-medication pain relief remedies. For example, applying cold packs or compresses for 20 – 30 minutes several times a day to the joint affected can lessen the inflammation and help ease the pain. Elevating the affected joint on a pillow and resting will also help in reducing the pain. Again, drinking water will help in stabilizing the uric acid level to a normal level.

There are several natural remedies for treating gout at home. These include organic apple cider vinegar, baking soda, cherries, bromelain, beet juice and exercise.[13]

The organic apple cider vinegar is known to provide up to 90% pain relief within one to two days. To use this method of pain relief, mix one to two tablespoons of the vinegar with eight ounces of water. Once mixed, it can be drank all at once or sipped over a period of time. It is recommended to try both methods and to determine which method is most effective.

Another option for pain relief involves using the baking soda. To do so, mix eight ounces of water and mix it with one-half of a teaspoon of baking soda. It is important to drink this in one sitting; however, one may need to drink up to six glasses per day for one to two days before pain relief occurs. In some cases the first glass of the mixture may provide immediate pain relief. It is important to note that baking soda may increase blood pressure so this method may not be a good remedy for those that suffer from hypertension.

As discussed earlier, consumption of cherries can reduce the levels of uric acid in the body. A study confirmed that eating ten to twelve cherries a day reduced gout attacks by 35% and consuming up to three servings over two days reduced them by 50%.

Bromelain is a mix of a number of different protein digesting enzymes. Further, it is a natural blood thinner and anti-inflammatory that also promotes blood circulation by blocking the production of compounds that cause swelling and pain. In 1957, Ralph Heinicke, a Dole Pineapple Company chemist, discovered that pineapple stems contained high levels of this natural remedy. Pineapples are the only known fruit to contain Bromelain. Since the Bromelain is found in the stem of the pineapple it is important to take it in the form of a capsule, tablet or powder rather than just eating the fruit itself. Throughout a gout attack, take 500mg of this capsule every three hours to aid in the breakdown of the crystal-like deposits causing the attack. In order to prevent future attacks, take the same dosage twice a day on an empty stomach along with 500mg of quercentin.[14]

According to the Centers for disease Control and Prevention, adults should exercise for at least 30 minutes per day at a moderate intensity level most days throughout the week. This regime is known to help with the prevention of gout and also helps in reducing the intensity of the attacks. It is important to note that the exercise should not be performed during an attack. Once an attack has passed, the exercise regimen should be started back up slowly.[15]

For those suffering from gout it is important that their loved ones and caregivers have a good understand of the disease, the things that can prevent recurrences and the things that can help ease the symptoms during an attack.